The Medical Job Interview

THE MEDICAL JOB INTERVIEW

Secrets for Success

Colin John Mumford

BMedSci, BM, BS, DM, FRCP Edin
Dip IMC RCSEd
Consultant Neurologist
Department of Clinical Neurosciences
Western General Hospital
Edinburgh

Blackwell
Science

© 2000 by
Blackwell Science Ltd
Editorial Offices:
Osney Mead, Oxford OX2 0EL
25 John Street, London WC 1N 2BS
23 Ainslie Place, Edinburgh EH3 6AJ
350 Main Street, Malden
  MA 02148 5018, USA
54 University Street, Carlton
  Victoria 3053, Australia
10, rue Casimir Delavigne
  75006 Paris, France

Other Editorial Offices:
Blackwell Wissenschafts-Verlag GmbH
Kurfürstendamm 57
10707 Berlin, Germany

Blackwell Science KK
MG Kodenmacho Building
7–10 Kodenmacho Nihombashi
Chuo-ku, Tokyo 104, Japan

Iowa State University Press
A Blackwell Science Company
2121 S. State Avenue
Ames, Iowa 50014-8300, USA

The right of the Author to be
identified as the Author of this Work
has been asserted in accordance
with the Copyright, Designs and
Patents Act 1988.

First published 2000
Reprinted 2001 (twice), 2002

Set by BookEns Ltd, Royston, Herts
Printed and bound in Great Britain
at the Alden Press, Oxford

The Blackwell Science logo is a
trade mark of Blackwell Science Ltd,
registered at the United Kingdom
Trade Marks Registry

DISTRIBUTORS

Marston Book Services Ltd
PO Box 269
Abingdon, Oxon OX14 4YN
(*Orders:* Tel: 01235 465500
     Fax: 01235 465555)

The Americas
Blackwell Publishing
c/o AIDC
PO Box 20
50 Winter Sport Lane
Williston, VT 05495-0020
(*Orders:* Tel: 800 216 2522
     Fax: 802 864 7626)

Canada
Login Brothers Book Company
324 Saulteaux Crescent
Winnipeg, Manitoba R3J 3T2
(*Orders:* Tel: 204 837 2987)

Australia
Blackwell Science Pty Ltd
54 University Street
Carlton, Victoria 3053
(*Orders:* Tel: 3 9347 0300
     Fax: 3 9347 5001)

A catalogue record for this title
is available from the British Library

ISBN 0-632-05527-8

Library of Congress
Cataloguing-in-publication Data

Mumford, Colin John
  The medical job interview: secrets
  of success/Colin John Mumford
    p. cm.
  Includes index.
  ISBN 0-632-05527-8
  1. Medical personnel—interviews.
  2. Employment interviewing.
  3. Physicians—Employment.
  4. Medicine—Vocational guidance.
  I. Title. [DNLM: 1. Interview. 2.
Job Application.
W 21 M962m 2000]

For further information on
Blackwell Science, visit our website:
www.blackwell-science.com

CONTENTS

Contents

INTRODUCTION

The aim of this short book is simple. It is to make you successful in your next medical job interview. It is quite possible to be a wonderful medical student or doctor with encyclopaedic knowledge of medical conditions, first-class clinical skills and a wonderful rapport with all your patients, but if you can't perform well in a job interview then you will get nowhere. This book sets out to give you tips that will be equally relevant, whether you are a final-year medical student applying for your first house job, a senior house officer trying to break through on to the specialist registrar career ladder, or if you are reaching the end of your specialist registrar training and are seeking appointment to your first consultant post.

Note that this book is written for the UK system of medical training. Graduates in Ireland and western Europe may find some of the information given useful. However, I must leave it up to colleagues in the USA and Canada to decide whether they feel that this 'very British approach' can win over interview panels in North America!

Even British graduates need to appreciate that I am giving advice from the point of view of a hospital consultant who has worked his way up through the British *hospital* medical career ladder. A rather different emphasis and series of tricks are needed for breaking into the world of general practice. All the same, some of the tips given here may be a useful start for someone approaching an interview to become a registrar in general practice, or even seeking appointment to their first post as principal in general practice.

The astonishing thing about most British medical graduates is that although they prepare in enormous detail for clinical medical school exams and for postgraduate diplomas, such as the MRCP(UK), MRCOG, FRCS and so on, most of them put relatively little thought into planning their strategy for handling a medical job interview. This is a grave error since there is no doubt that good interview technique can be learned. Some people begin their careers already good at it, but others are so bad that they could be described as appalling in an interview and it is this latter group who most need to do their homework prior to facing an interview panel!

Throughout this book I've tended to use the word 'he' when, of course, I mean 'he or she'. Writing 'he or she' every time becomes clumsy.

BEFORE THE INTERVIEW

chapter 2

SPOTTING THE ADVERT

It sounds ridiculous, but some individuals fail at the very first hurdle in their efforts to climb the medical career ladder and that is because they fail to spot the advert for the job which they want. This is a catastrophic mistake since the one way to guarantee not being short listed is not to apply for the job in the first place. Therefore, as soon as you are even contemplating applying for your next move up the medical ladder you should be scrutinizing the relevant medical press to see which adverts are appearing, what sort of jobs are available and starting to focus your mind on the locations where you would most like to work. This may mean remaining in your current geographical area, or you may have a particular desire to move to a different part of the country for your next job.

In general terms this task is made easy for British graduates because the classified section of the *British Medical Journal* lists all the available jobs coming up and these are conveniently grouped under headings according to speciality. Remember, however, that editors and typesetters of the *British Medical Journal* are human and it is not uncommon to see an advert for a post, say, in neurology, advertised in error under the section headed neurosurgery. Occasionally, hospitals perform rather underhand tricks and – for reasons best known to themselves – may decide to place an advert in a not-very-obvious location which may be in a national newspaper, in the back pages of a weekly free journal such as *Hospital Doctor*, or in some other obscure location.

If you think that a post is about to be advertised yet are struggling to find the actual advertisement, then you could phone the appropriate personnel or medical staffing department at the relevant hospital or regional postgraduate centre and asking when the particular post will be coming up. Expressing such enthusiasm at an early stage does no harm at all.

One word of caution is required at this point and that is that some individuals are uncertain whether or not they should apply for a job. This is particularly true at the start of a medical career when people are not sure if they should hold out for 'the best' pre-registration house officer job, or whether they should accept something 'second-rate'. Equally, this is particularly acute at the end of the medical ladder when senior specialist registrars are uncertain whether a 'plum consultant post' is about to come up, or whether they should go for a post which they might consider 'second division'. The way to decide whether to apply or not is to ask yourself that, if you eventually get through to the medical interview and find yourself successful 'will I stand up, punch the air and shout "Yahooo!" '? If you are uncertain as to whether you would be able to express such overt enthusiasm then you probably should not be applying for the post at all. This rule is there to be broken, however, and if you are genuinely not sure whether a job is the right one for you then there is no harm in putting in an application and at least going part-way through the selection process, provided that you withdraw before you find yourself sitting in the interview. You can withdraw, if necessary, on the morning of the interview but it is a complete 'no no' to sit in an interview, be offered the job and then reject the offer following the interview. This goes down extremely badly with interview panels and will land you with an undesirable reputation. On the other hand, a cautious application and polite, tactful withdrawal prior to the interview, with careful explanation to the relevant consultants, will not usually cause too much upset.

'THE COMMANDO OPERATION' TO GET ON THE SHORT LIST

Once you have seen the correct advert for you, the next steps, which include submitting the application, preparing your curriculum vitae (CV) and making sure you get on the short list, can best be thought of as a 'commando operation'. Royal Marine commandos are enormously successful at what they do, basically because they leave no margin for error. Every item of equipment is checked, rechecked and tested in enormous detail. If you seriously want to be successful in the medical job interview then you need to begin a thorough, almost military, operation to make absolutely sure that you get the job. Like it or not, job interviews are competitive and accordingly you have to show the interview panel that you are better than everybody else that has made an application for the post. Since some jobs may receive in excess of 200 applicants, if you sit back and wait to be short listed you can guarantee that you will simply be a 'face in the crowd' and you are very unlikely to be short listed unless there is something extraordinarily unusual about your CV.

Therefore, as soon as the appropriate job advert appears you need to be on the phone getting the relevant application forms and you need to start preparing your CV. The application forms will almost certainly give you information about the hospital, including names of relevant consultants and appropriate contact phone numbers.

Your immediate goal following receipt of the job description is to get yourself on to the short list. Other people can help you with this. Indeed, a well-judged phone call from one of your current consultants to his friend or golfing partner, who is a consultant in the relevant hospital, can work wonders. You may feel that it is somehow underhand to ask your consultant to make a phone call on your behalf, but, unfortunately, some of your competitors will have done this and you need to make sure you are playing in the same ball game. Bear in mind that although a helpful phone call putting forward your name may significantly improve your chances of getting on to the short list, once you are on the short list you are on your own and it is very unlikely that persuasive words from one of your senior colleagues will actually make a difference in the interview itself.

TO VISIT OR NOT TO VISIT?

Many candidates wonder if it is 'worthwhile' visiting the relevant hospital before the short list is announced. Anybody that does not visit the hospital is, in my view, significantly reducing their chance of getting placed on the short list. There is no doubt that a voluntary visit, made early and at your own expense, in order to look around wards, departments, X-ray facilities and so on — and ideally to meet one or two of the consultants — can be enormously rewarding. The progress of a whole career can be changed by 'bumping into' the relevant consultant or professor in the corridor outside his office. If you can achieve this then you are already one rung higher than all your competitors in the fight to get on to the short list. Be mindful of the fact that most senior consultants are very busy and do not take kindly to being interrupted in their office, or being stopped whilst walking in the corridor outside their office. Therefore, you need to be sharp and to the point in introducing yourself to the consultant and asking if there is a point 'later in the day' when you might be able to spend 5 minutes with him since you are 'most interested' in the forthcoming job on his unit. Most consultants will accept this sort of approach but will not wish to spend 5 or 10 minutes in the corridor discussing things when they, undoubtedly, will have more important things to do. However, a request to meet later in the day may be acceptable to them.

If, having 'bumped into' the relevant consultant and he is not willing to see you, there is no reason at all why you shouldn't go and see his secretary and ask if you might talk to the consultant on another occasion, or whether there are a few moments at the end of the day when he will be less busy. If nothing else, you can attempt to endear yourself to the secretary who then may make a favourable comment later in the day when dealing with other aspects of the consultant's work.

This initial visit must not be confused with the visits which are frequently made following the publication of the short list. Many hospitals send a letter with their initial information pack saying something of along the lines of 'short listed candidates are invited to visit the hospital'. These visits will often be arranged and timetabled by the secretary of the most senior consultant involved and the hospital will reimburse you with the costs of your travel. Bear in mind that you will only have the chance of doing this once you are already on the short list and therefore a visit prior to short listing is, in my opinion, essential to show enthusiasm and to start to set yourself apart from the crowd.

The process of short listing will usually be done by the head of the relevant department to which you are applying and also a by a number of his consultant colleagues. It is very unlikely that members of the hospital management will be involved in the short listing process, although occasionally representatives of the regional postgraduate dean may have some votes in this process. Therefore, if you are going to make a visit prior to short listing and I advise that you do, concentrate solely on seeing the clinicians for whom you will be working. If the post which you are applying for is at junior house officer (JHO) or senior house officer (SHO) level, then try to see some of the specialist registrars working on the unit as well, since you would be surprised how much exchange of ideas takes place at the end of a ward round when consultants discuss with their registrars potential candidates for short listing.

Although the initial visit which I am advising prior to short listing could be considered as being 'relatively informal' you need all the while to be aware of the fact that you have one goal only and that is to convince the people whom you meet that you are the single best candidate for the forthcoming job. Accordingly, part of the process requires that you look smart, engage in appropriately focused conversation with the doctors you meet and, above all, have a large number of spare copies of your CV to distribute. Most of the senior clinicians will not have seen your CV until very shortly before they are asked to produce a short list so if your name is to be remembered, you must pull a CV out of your bag and leave it with the relevant consultant 'for perusal once you are gone'.

Once you have returned to your base hospital following this pre-short listing visit, make sure that you discuss what went on with your current bosses since if they have not already telephoned their colleagues at the new hospital to put in a word on your behalf, this is the time you should ask them to do so.

WHOM TO SEE ONCE YOU ARE SHORT LISTED

Once the short list has been produced and, hopefully, has your name on it, then whether or not you have previously visited you are now absolutely obliged to go and visit the relevant hospital. Generally speaking, your travel expenses for a visit at this stage will be refunded to you. Your priority, once again, is to meet with the consultants for whom you will be working, or, if a senior post, whom you will be working alongside, but bear in mind that during the interview itself there will almost certainly be some non-medical interviewers, for example, a member of the hospital management or a representative of the Trust Board. Therefore, at least one of your visits must be to the chief executive of the hospital, or, if not available, one of his senior management team. The reason for this is that you must be briefed regarding forthcoming developments in the hospital, be they new buildings, new clinics or a new approach to the delivery of medical care to the local community. You can gain a great deal of information by talking to senior managers and much of this information may not be known to the consultant staff who will be interviewing you. Having learned top quality and up-to-date information from the managers, you can sound highly impressive by discussing the way in which the hospital is going to evolve during the next few years and how you feel that you, as SHO, specialist registrar or consultant, will contribute to 'this blossoming service'. Additionally, and particularly if you are applying for a post at relatively senior level, make sure that you meet one or two consultants from related specialities. So, for example, if you are going for a post in cardiology then ensure you meet some of the cardiac surgeons. If you are applying for a post as a transplant surgeon, then the medical nephrologists and hepatologists would almost certainly be flattered if you took the trouble to meet them prior to the interview. Do not underestimate how much potential candidates are discussed over the table in the consultants' dining room and if your name is mentioned favourably here, it can work wonders in the final reckoning.

GETTING THE CURRICULUM VITAE RIGHT

Entire books are devoted to the right and wrong way to present a CV (sometimes called a 'résumé' by our colleagues in North America). Many formats are acceptable, but the document which is presented must look in pristine condition. It must be laser printed and laid out in a simple, readily accessible format. Make sure that the typing is broadly spaced and that dates describing the time spent in previous posts are clearly laid out. Modern interview panels take great pains to ensure that candidates have done the appropriate amount of general professional training and specialist training, and this is usually done right at the start of the interview. Watching a member of the interview panel struggling to piece together information from a poorly set out CV is desperately embarrassing and generally means rapid failure for the guilty candidate.

Most medical CVs are set out in a certain order, usually starting with personal details, education, medical degrees, medical diplomas and higher quali-fications, as well as a word about registration with the General Medical Council and membership of a med-ical defence organization. The CV should then describe your present and previous occupations. At some point in their careers most doctors usually decide to start with 'present appointment' and then work backwards in time. This is the strategy which I would advise. Remember to make your present appointment sound as attractive as possible; for example, you may think that you are simply 'spe-cialist registrar in general medicine', but if you think carefully you may find that you are also an honorary lecturer in medicine of the relevant university, or at least a clinical tutor to one or more medical students. All of these facets of your present appointment should be clearly stated.

When describing previous appointments, above all make sure that the dates between which each post was held are clearly set out. List the names of the consultants for whom you worked. If you have performed locum posts try and fit these in chronological order. If there are unexpected gaps in the sequence of dates running backwards in time then put in a comment to explain what was done during that vacant period of time.

Once you have dealt with present and previous posts in your CV, most interview panels then like to see other short sections describing your experience in your chosen speciality, teaching experience, management experience and, of course, a detailed description of research work which you have done. If you are applying for a relatively senior post it is likely that you will have written a number of publications and these should be presented in detail. Traditionally, work is presented in the following order: books, chapters in books, refereed papers, review articles, invited editorials, published abstracts of communications to learned societies, published correspondence, poster presentations and then any non-medical publications which you may have. You should conclude your CV by incorporating a section on your career development aims, other relevant information and a short section on your interests and hobbies. The final page should be a list of referees.

HOW TO CHOOSE A WINNING REFEREE

Selection of referees is not as immediately simple as it may seem. Your priority must be to get people who will say nice things about you. However, some referees are all too willing to give a reference which is remarkably mediocre and does not make you stand out in comparison with the competition. Therefore, you need to go and speak to your potential referees and be prepared to ask them outright if they would be willing to write a *good* reference for you. This may seem to be a rather pushy approach but there is no doubt that some senior medical staff will willingly agree to be a referee and then write rather uninspired comments which look bad when it comes to the interview. Short matter-of-fact references never help anybody. So feel free to ask your potential referee if they would be willing to write a detailed reference, outlining your good points and explaining the reasons why you would be very suitable for the post which you are proposing to apply for. Also do not hesitate about choosing a larger number of referees than was specifically requested in the job description and advertisement. I advise people that if the request is for two references then the names of three referees should be given. If the request is for three referees then four names should be offered. One reason for this is that hospitals may request references at very short notice and sometimes referees are away or abroad. Failure to produce a reference is a total catastrophe. You must therefore offer the names of 'stand-by' referees. Moreover, many personnel departments will simply seek a reference from all of the names given as potential referees without thinking how many they originally specified. If an interview panel is deluged with a large number of strongly worded, glowing references speaking about you in the highest possible terms, then this can do nothing but good. Remember to make sure that you give the phone number and probably also the fax numbers and e-mail addresses of your referees, in case details are requested at very short notice.

THE INTERVIEW

chapter 3

WHERE, WHEN AND HOW

If you have followed the advice in the first part of this book then with luck you will have made it to the short list and accordingly you will be invited to attend for interview. Like so many aspects of getting on in a medical career, preparation for the interview needs to start even before you receive the letter inviting you to attend. Remember that you are not such an important candidate that the date, time or location of the interview will be changed just to suit you. Therefore, it is perfectly reasonable, when applying for a job, to ask the hospital personnel department if a date has already been set for the interview and you should ensure that you are not on holiday or out of the country for another reason on the allotted date. Only under very exceptional circumstances will you be able to persuade an interview panel to change the date of an interview and this is only likely to happen for very senior appointments if you are clearly the front-running candidate.

The second vital issue which sounds obvious but which is frequently a stumbling block for junior doctors is the need to find out exactly the location of the interview. This is not as simple as it may seem since frequently candidates assume that the interview will take place in the hospital at which they have applied for a job, whereas in fact the interview is held at the regional postgraduate centre, the Trust Board offices or the headquarters of the regional health authority. All these are traps for the unwary and if this sort of elementary information is not sorted out at an early stage you will be rattled if you eventually do make it to the interview. There is nothing worse than turning up a few minutes late for an interview and having to apologise that you are late because you went to the wrong venue. Under no circumstances whatsoever should you be late for the interview. To turn up late implies a degree of shoddy planning which will immediately alienate most senior doctors, who will think that if you are incapable of getting to an interview on time, that there is no chance you would actually make it to their clinic or to their ward rounds on time.

It is perfectly reasonable to try and find out who will be interviewing you. Sometimes for posts at junior house doctor (JHO) or senior house doctor (SHO) level this may be a panel as small as two individuals. More frequently the panel is much larger than that and for most specialist registrar appointments, and certainly for consultant grade appointments, the panel may be as big as 11 or 12 people. The reason for this is that most interview panels are now convened to a relatively set formula. There will be representatives of the consultants for whom you are going to be working, of course, but, in addition, there will be representatives of the relevant university, somebody representing the regional postgraduate dean and a member of the hospital Trust Board. Bear in mind that this latter individual may know very little about medicine and, indeed, may know little about the day-to-day workings of a hospital. This individual is sometimes jokingly referred to using the generic term, 'the vicar's wife'. He may ask some very unexpected questions and it is worth being well prepared for the questions which may come from 'the vicar's wife', about which more later.

Note also that for specialist registrar and consultant appointments there will be another important individual who will be the Royal College representative, sometimes referred to as the 'national panellist' for interviews in Scotland. These members of the panel have a slightly different remit in that they are there not to assess who is best for the job, but simply to ensure that every candidate who attends for the interview has done the required amount of previous training, for example, general professional training before specialization and this member of the panel confirms with the chairman of the interview panel that you are 'suitable for appointment to the offered post'.

Remember also that although you may have spent many hours trying to 'bump into' the professor and head of department in the corridor outside his office, whilst he will almost certainly be on the panel, he is not usually the chairman. The chairman of large interview panels is frequently a consultant from a different speciality and sometimes from a different hospital. Alternatively, he may be the medical director of the hospital in which you are applying to work. The chairman of the panel is there to ensure fair play and may not, in fact, have a vote in the final judgement as to who is appointed.

Knowing the individual members of the panel in advance can be enormously helpful in being successful in the medical job interview. Once you have heard that you are short listed you should contact the relevant personnel department and ask if they are able to let you know the composition of the panel. Some hospitals are rather cagey about this, believing it is somehow 'unfair', but in general terms most personnel departments are willing to give you a list and job titles of the people comprising the panel. You should then find out exactly who they are, where they work and what they do. If you have not already met them on a previous visit then you may wish to make a further visit to ensure that your face is known to as many members of the panel as possible.

The interview itself is likely to be held in a large, relatively formal, room. Many hospitals have a 'boardroom' which they reserve almost exclusively for this purpose. In the same way that you must know exactly the geographical location of the interview building, you must also make absolutely sure that you can find your way to the correct room. Shrewd candidates also make careful note of the nearest toilet.

WHAT TO WEAR

Clothing for an interview is largely a matter of personal choice but nevertheless the concept of 'power dressing' should be adhered to as far as possible. Whatever you select from your wardrobe, your goal must be to look entirely professional and 101% appropriate for the post for which you are applying. Most senior hospital physicians are relatively conservative people in the way that they dress and they will expect you to do likewise. For men a dark suit with a pristine white shirt and appropriate contrasting tie is undoubtedly the most appropriate. Your shoes must be gleaming. Men should not wear any obvious jewellery simply because it runs the risk of alienating one or more members of the panel. You may, of course, wear a discreet tie clip and appropriate, unobtrusive cuff-links.

The choice of tie can be all important. Indeed, if you are forced into the 'uniform' of a dark suit and a white shirt, then the choice of a good tie is one of the few ways in which you can display some individuality. The tie should be of a pattern best described as 'classic'. For example, woven silk or plain silk with a simple pattern. Sometimes relatively bright colours including red, orange and bright yellow can look quite striking and yet, at the same time, retain a feeling of great professionalism. I would urge caution against wearing any sort of club tie. Even if you happen to know that the head of department was in the same Royal Air Force squadron as your father, it is ill-advised to wear the appropriate club or regimental tie since you run the risk of being questioned about the tie and its significance. One of two things will then happen: either you will be able to answer in a very erudite manner impressing the former Group Captain on the interview panel and this will alienate the other members of the panel; or, alternatively, you will not be able to answer the probing questions relating to the provenance of your tie and you will then look totally ridiculous.

Clothing for women is altogether more difficult and it is quite reasonable to ask for advice from senior female medical colleagues. A suit or sober dress is entirely reasonable. Whatever you choose, think all the time that the guiding principle must be to appear totally professional.

One word on smell and that is 'don't'. Excessive use of cosmetics is also to be avoided. Female candidates may, of course, apply make-up but it should be done in a manner that gives a professional air without looking garish. Small items of jewellery are also quite reasonable for women. In the same way that men should avoid jewellery, they should also avoid anything other than minimal application of aftershave. Most panels will object to what they perceive as a 'man wearing perfume'.

HOW TO SIT

It is possible to anticipate what will happen when you are called into the interview room. You will be sitting outside the room usually with other candidates, most of whom will not be engaging in conversation with you. When your name is called you need to stand up smartly and follow the invitation to enter the interview room. First impressions are all important and you need, as you go through the door, firstly to look professional, secondly to look interested in what is going on and thirdly – and above all – to start giving an immediate impression that you are the only suitable candidate for the job. One way to achieve this is to acknowledge as many of the interview panel as is possible at least with eye contact and perhaps a small nod. If the panel is very large this will not be possible. Do not look at the floor or stare blankly at the wall behind the chairman of the panel. Do not sit down until you are invited to do so.

When you do sit, try and avoid giving the impression of a captured soldier undergoing interrogation. It is reasonable to turn the chair to a slight angle and to sit with your legs crossed if you wish with your hands on your lap. Try to avoid looking terrified or gripping the arms of the chair tightly. Do not, under any circumstances, adopt a posture that could be regarded as 'slouching'. If the chair is a relatively comfy chair with a low back this can be difficult and you may wish to sit forward on the edge of the chair. The overriding goal is to give an air of cool professionalism.

EYE CONTACT, WHERE TO LOOK AND THE 'CURRICULUM VITAE RUN-THROUGH'

Virtually all medical job interviews begin the same way and that is that the chairman of the panel will introduce you to all the other members of the panel. Frequently you will know these individuals since you may have been working with them already, or you may have recently had lengthy discussions with them regarding the reasons why you want the job. No matter how well you know the panel you must 'play a straight bat' from this point onwards. It may be the case that somebody interviewing you is one of your regular drinking or mountaineering partners, but this fact will not be known to other members of the panel and excessive informality simply goes down very badly. An interview is a formal occasion and you must behave appropriately. Therefore, when each member of the panel is introduced it is reasonable to nod and say 'hello', but probably no more than that. Once the introductions are completed the chairman of the interview panel will almost certainly hand straight over to the representative of the Royal College or the national panellist, or, alternatively, another member of the panel who will start going through your curriculum vitae.

Bear in mind at this point that although every word of your CV is known to you and you may be able to recite it verbatim, it is possible that the panel member now holding your CV may never have seen it before. So, although you may think it is obvious that your career progression during the past 6 years is written down with impeccable clarity, the person now looking at your hieroglyphics may not find it quite so clear. You need to nod and make small comments of agreement as this panel member starts going through your CV noting where you went to school, where you trained, where you did your house jobs, where you did your SHO rotation and so on.

While this panel member is doing this task, he is totting up in his head the number of months you have spent in each job, basically satisfying himself that you have done the right amount of previous training to be suitable for the present post. Frequently this adding up procedure goes wrong and it is perfectly reasonable for you to politely interrupt and correct the panel member if the sums are going awry. Be ready at this point to have answers to questions regarding what you did during any obvious gaps in your professional training. You may think that your CV clearly indicates the 4 months that you spent at a mission hospital in central Africa, but it may not be immediately evident to the Royal College representative struggling to find his way around your CV and you need to be ready to help if necessary. Try to avoid getting into lengthy discussions regarding what you have or have not done in the past at this point, since this early part of the interview is very much an assessment to check that you are suitable for the job in question. Also, be absolutely certain that you can recall every detail of your own training progression since candidates that struggle to remember exactly where they did their first SHO job can look very silly indeed in front of interview panels.

Once this initial 'CV run-through' has been completed the chairman of the interview panel will invite other members of the panel to question you in turn. It is possible that not all the members of the interview panel will ask questions. The actual questions which you may be asked are considered in the next section of this book, but in starting to consider how to deal with the questions two general principles apply. The first of these is that whatever question you are asked you must try to give your answers promptly, brightly and using the guiding principle of 'cool professionalism with sparkle'. Your style of answering should be confident, polite, to the point and yet not bland. A brief reflective moment to gather your thoughts before you start to speak is fine, but avoid absolutely any prolonged 'pregnant pauses'. Remember that although this interview is the most important thing that has happened to you for many months, for the members of the panel it may be something of a chore and you may be the eighth candidate that they have interviewed that afternoon. Therefore, a degree of enthusiasm and sparkle must come through in all your answers to draw the attention of the panel to you and to gain their interest.

The second guiding principle of answering interview questions is related and is this: although just one member of the panel will have asked you the question, you need to deliver your answer to all the members of the panel. In other words, although you should start by facing the questioner and beginning your answer, as you develop your answer you should engage in eye contact with other members of the panel, turning your head if necessary, to make sure that the right side of the room is not bored if the question came from the left side of the panel and vice versa. Your goal is to impress not just the person who has asked you the question but to make sure that you win over every member of the panel with every answer to every question. The art of head turning and gaining eye contact with others is not one which doctors practise. Watch politicians delivering a speech to a large audience. They do it well. That is because they have been trained and it is quite reasonable for you to train yourself by asking some friends to give you a mock interview. If there are two or three of them make them sit in different areas of the room and practise getting all of them involved with your answers to their questions.

GESTURE

Many interview candidates sit with their hands firmly clasped together or, worse still, their arms folded throughout the whole interview. This is a disaster and gives a very bad impression to the panel. Again, observe a politician being interviewed on television; watch how they use their hands. Seldom is there any wild, expansive gesture, but very frequently there is small reinforcement of points that they are making by using small gestures with one hand. This is something which you should practise. Also, panels are very impressed with a reasoned answer containing several components, each thread of which is enumerated by tapping one finger on to the fingers of the opposite hand as though you were counting. Simple gesture makes for a good delivery and can be surprisingly good at making one candidate 'stand out from the crowd'. Gesture should be subtle and restrained but should be used. Just be careful not to overdo it to turn the whole thing into a game of charades.

HOW TO END THE INTERVIEW

When the interview is over and all the questions have been asked then you will be invited to leave. This instruction may be preceded by the chairman of the panel letting you know that they will come to a decision perhaps later that day, in which case he may invite you to wait. Alternatively, the chairman may suggest that the decision will not be made until the following day, in which case you will be asked if the secretary of the panel has got appropriate contact details for you. Make up your mind in advance whether you are going to stay to hear the result, if it is only going to be an hour or so later. In general terms interview panels like to be able to greet the successful candidate at the end of the afternoon, so stay if you can. However, if you have travelled a long distance and have a train or plane to catch to return home, then they will not be irritated if you ask them to contact you by telephone with news of the outcome.

When you stand from your chair do not blindly walk out of the room but make a point of acknowledging as many members of the panel as possible with a small nod and the single word, 'thank you', addressed to the panel as a whole. Then leave, trying to ensure that you know which way the door of the interview room opens to avoid unnecessary pulling when you should be pushing. You must also make absolutely certain that you do not use the wrong door and unintentionally exit into the broom cupboard, thus generating an embarrassing scene with any pretence of 'cool professionalism' being irretrievably lost.

THE QUESTIONS

One very important mistake that interview candidates make is that they fail to realize that it is entirely feasible to work out what questions you will be asked in the interview long before you ever find yourself sitting in front of the panel. Many candidates do not believe that such a feat is possible. However, the sequence of questions which is asked in a medical job interview, particularly when interviewing candidates for senior house officer (SHO) and specialist registrar posts, is remarkably consistent. To some extent the flow of questions which a candidate will be asked when applying for a consultant-grade job can also be largely anticipated in advance. In other words, some questions are inevitable.

INEVITABLE QUESTIONS

With some thought it is very easy to see what the 'inevitable' questions will be. If, for example, you are applying to be a specialist registrar in gastro-enterology in a major city in the Midlands then you will undoubtedly be asked, firstly, 'why gastro-enterology?' and, secondly, 'why this city'? Whether you like the thought of these questions or not you are under an absolute obligation to have clear, well thought out and concise answers to both these questions. Remember when you frame your answers that all the time the essence is not just to show that you are good at answering these questions, the overwhelming priority is to show through your answers that you are unequivocally the best person for the job. Any sort of rambling or waffling answer to these first questions, for example, comments such as 'well, I'm really not sure what I want to do, but I think gastroenterology seems like a good idea' is a recipe for disaster. Equally, when considering the city in which you have applied to work, remember that the unit in that city may have been the product of years and years of work by the members of the panel who are now interviewing you and comments such as 'well, I thought I'd try here first because the advert was the first to appear in the *BMJ*, but I'm equally enthusiastic about cities X and Y' is not the sort of answer that builds up warmth between the interview panel and you.

You need to frame and construct your answers with some care and it would be my suggestion that you adhere to the guiding principle suggested in Chapter 3 of this book, which could loosely be described as 'cool professionalism with enthusiasm'. You must show that: firstly, you are perfectly capable as a doctor; secondly, that you will be capable of performing brilliantly in the post which is on offer and; thirdly, demonstrate that you are entirely professional about all you do. However, your answers must have a certain gloss — a kind of sparkle — which demonstrates an enthusiasm which is often not shown by the candidates against whom you will be competing. Therefore, let 'cool professionalism with enthusiasm' be in the back of your mind whilst you are delivering your answers.

Remember that the interview panel will like to feel that some praise is being offered for their unit through the medium of your answers. Therefore, a good answer dealing with the question 'why do you want to come to this city?' might include observations such as 'you have to look a long way to find a training programme in gastroenterology which is as well constructed and offers such good variety as the post in this city. There are very few other centres that allow a rotation between hospitals giving me a chance to work with a number of different consultants in the field, all of whom have differing sub-speciality interests'.

You can then add other riders to your comments according to the particular circumstances of the post for which you have applied, for example, 'of particular appeal in the present post is the close liaison which you enjoy with (for instance) the regional liver transplant programme, since this is an area of gastroenterology that particularly interests me'. Or you might add, for example, 'the present post is particularly exciting because of the high intensity emergency work which is done and the close links which you have with the supra-regional trauma centre which is on this site'. All the time your answers must be focused and enthusiastic, making it quite plain that no other job is the one for you except for the present job which is on offer.

It is only in interviews at a relatively junior level that you can expect to be asked 'why this subject?' and, again, your answers must be well thought out and show total enthusiasm and commitment to the speciality which you are trying to enter.

A word of caution is necessary at this point for the candidate who is applying for an SHO, specialist registrar, or even a consultant job in a location in which he is already working. In Chapter 3, I have drawn attention to the grave risk that candidates who are well known to the panel will be excessively informal and sometimes even flippant with an interview panel whom they already know well. This is a great mistake and is to be avoided at all costs. This scenario also gives rise to a question which may floor an unwary candidate and that is something along the lines of 'surely, having worked with us for the past 12 months you cannot possibly want to carry on working with us for the next 5 or 6 years'? This sometimes comes as an unexpected question for a candidate and a clear answer, again avoiding inappropriate humour or flippancy, is necessary. My suggestion would be to turn the question on its head and use it to your advantage by saying something along the lines of 'it is precisely because I have had the opportunity of working in this department and with several members of the panel, that I realize exactly what an excellent opportunity for further training in gastroenterology this unit offers. I have had the opportunity to take part in the in-patient and out-patient service as well as helping to shape our present emergency service and I very much want to develop these aspects of the service in the next stage of my career'.

It would be perfectly reasonable to add (whether you believe it or not) 'indeed, having had the opportunity to compare my experience in this department with colleagues who have worked in other departments, I can see that there are few other departments around the country that can offer (for example) a specialist registrar position with so many exciting opportunities as the present post'. And you could conclude this rather difficult moment in the interview by reinforcing the point 'so it is *because* I am already familiar with the department that I am so excited and enthusiastic about the present post which is on offer'.

PROBABLE QUESTIONS

Some of the questions which are listed above can be guaranteed to be asked in just about every medical interview. There will then follow a series of questions which can also largely be anticipated. If you are applying for a post at a junior level you will be asked about your experience of the clinical training course in your medical school, how much time you spent in general medicine, general surgery, accident and emergency and so on. Most interview panellists who will be genuinely interested in the medical curricula at other medical schools may well ask a question along the lines of 'if you were planning your own medical curriculum what would you alter'? There is no right or wrong answer to this but a thoughtful answer which makes sense to the interview panellist will usually go down well.

In framing an answer to this sort of a question you should be prepared to provoke a little discussion with the panel and don't worry if they seem to disagree with some of your observations; stick to your guns and say why you would change the curriculum in the way that you have proposed. The only wrong way to answer the question is to spend a long time 'umming' and 'aaahing' and then say something rather limp like 'well I thought our course was probably alright, I don't think anything needs changing'. This sort of answer loses the feeling of enthusiasm which you are trying to convey.

Again, if you are applying for a post at a relatively junior level you can be certain that some time will be spent asking about your elective period. Be sure that you know exactly where you went and if you worked with anybody famous, who they were, since it is possible that they will be known to the panel. Conversely, if you went somewhere exotic, for example, the Caribbean and spent the whole 8-week period playing golf, lying on the beach and windsurfing, then do not say this in your answer. Whilst many interview panels will realize that this is a very important part of student elective periods, they will not wish to be told so in the formal environment of an interview and you must therefore be prepared to talk about the difficulties of delivering community paediatric care in remote areas of Caribbean islands or something similar. Remember that you are showing 'cool professionalism' all the time. Whilst one or two members of the panel may, themselves, be enthusiastic golfers or windsurfers, they will not wish to hear that this was the way in which you spent your elective period.

Research and publications are a guaranteed part of any interview. If you have had the skill to produce an undergraduate publication and you are applying for a junior house officer (JHO) or SHO job, then undergraduate publications greatly impress the panel and you may be surprised to be asked about this in some detail. Therefore, you must be able to quote the title of any papers which resulted from your work and you should have pre-prepared a short paragraph in your head which will explain in simple terms to individuals who are not familiar with your field, what you did and why your research was of interest. Remember at this point the 'vicar's wife' figure on the panel, in other words, remember that your answer must be intelligible to somebody that may not know any medicine at all. Sometimes interview candidates of both junior and senior level are quite incapable of explaining the nature of their research work in a simple way to people that are very familiar with medicine but not familiar with the specific area of research. If you cannot explain your own research in a simple way to an interview panel, then they will lose interest in your answer and at the same time that they lose interest in your answer, they will also lose interest in you.

It is worth stressing a third 'guiding principle' at this point and that is that many interview candidates believe it is up to them to show that 'they are right for the job'. Curiously, this is not necessarily the overriding goal in an interview because it could be argued that everybody that has found their way on to the short list is 'right for the job'. If they were not 'right for the job' then they would not have been short listed in the first place. So, another thought needs to be in the back of your mind as you are delivering all your answers in the interview and that is that you need to show the panel that 'not only are you right for the job, *but the job is right for you at this stage in your career'*. This assertion requires a little thought but it is very true that there is often little to choose between interview candidates who have been short listed for a given post and in the discussion which follows 'behind closed doors' after all candidates have been interviewed, a decision which may seem to be very difficult indeed can sometimes be resolved by the interview panel deciding the answer to the question 'for which of the candidates whom we have just interviewed is this job the most appropriate at this stage in their career'? Therefore, if you — when delivering your answers — have stressed the point that not only are you the right, most appropriate person for the job, but also that the job is clearly the right way that you 'should be moving' at this stage in your career progression, then that message may hit home and getting that point across is frequently the single best way to win over an interview panel. Panels do not like individuals who seem to be 'drifting' from one job to the next. They are far more impressed by an individual who has 'nailed their colours to the mast' and who has demonstrated a clear career direction. Part of that demonstration means that you need to show the panel that the job is right for you at this moment in time.

PROBLEM QUESTIONS

There are a number of 'sticky moments' which often crop up in interviews and rather surprisingly some of these can also be anticipated and a way out identified. It is often sensible to have identified the escape routes from these 'sticky' interview moments before you are faced with them in front of a formal panel. The following are some examples.

You haven't done any research

Most hospital specialists need to do research. Certainly, they need to have published a few papers before getting to senior level. Some individuals are wonderful clinicians and seem to get a long way up the career ladder without doing any research at all. The time this matters is when they are faced with an interview panel. If your CV is short on publications and original research, then you need to have some sort of an answer ready in case this issue is brought up. Rather than meekly admitting that you are a failure when it comes to writing papers, it is better to try and turn this shortcoming into a strength, perhaps by saying something like 'you will see from my CV that my greatest strengths are in the field of clinical medicine. My whole career so far has been very much orientated towards a clinical progression rather than a research or academic approach. I think my greatest contribution has been in liaison with my research colleagues and providing a source of patients and clinical ideas to enhance their own research. Therefore, I feel I have contributed to a number of different research projects over the years, but *as a clinician* and I have not been the major author of any of the resulting publications'. This may or may not be true but an answer along these lines is at least an attempt to turn a weakness into a strength.

You're applying for a 5-year rotation but the whole panel knows that you really want to go and work in Australia as soon as possible

Many junior doctors express enthusiasm to spend 1 or 2 years abroad at some point during their career and there is no need to hide this fact during the interview. The concern that worries interview panels most is if they think a new appointee is going to leave within a few months of arriving in a post since then a replacement will need to be found very quickly

and that does not go down well. You do not, however, need to keep the fact that you are thinking of
doing a year or two abroad a secret, but it is reasonable to give your overseas intentions a rather low
profile and to take an approach along the lines of
'although I have said for some time I would be
interested in exploring the possibility of working
overseas for a year or two, my major interest is to get
an excellent training in gastroenterology (for example) and the present post offers me the chance of
getting such a training. Therefore, my prime enthusiasm is to gain appointment to the present job and
work my way through this rotation for a number of
years. It may be that in years to come I may think
about exploring the possibility of a year abroad, but
that would only be with the full agreement of the
senior colleagues with whom I was working at that
time'.

You don't really want the job but your 'significant other' works in this city

Candidates are often surprised that interview panels
are remarkably human. Therefore, if you have
pressing social, domestic or family reasons why you
want to work in this city, it is quite acceptable to
say so. If you are a total 'no-hoper', then a plea that
your boyfriend or girlfriend lives and works in this
city is unlikely to secure you the job. However, if
you are running neck and neck with one of the
other candidates and you have a pressing domestic
reason why you would like to come to this particular city, then that is often influential when it
comes to decision time. Accordingly, you do not
need to be afraid of mentioning your social situation as one reason for wanting to work in a particular city. Comments in that regard, however, *must*
be linked with the sorts of answers offered in
paragraphs above, indicating a strong enthusiasm
for the post, the training which is offered, the

individuals with whom you would be working and so on.

It's far too early in your career for the job that you are applying for but you are 'chancing your arm'

This is a difficult issue and interview panels will often identify this problem very quickly. Occasionally, extreme enthusiasm and confidence both before and during the interview will win the day here. This problem is actually less frequent following the introduction of the Calman training system for specialist registrars in the UK, since this system now dictates that candidates must have done a certain amount of general professional training at SHO level before they are allowed to enter the specialist registrar grade and at the end of the specialist registrar period there is a strictly defined time period during which specialist registrars may start to look for their consultant job.

Nevertheless, it sometimes happens that a relatively junior SHO wants to apply for the perfect specialist registrar rotation in the very best centre and, in my view, it is quite reasonable to make every effort to get that job since the chance may not come around again for very many years. You must then be prepared to take a relatively aggressive stance in an interview making it quite plain that you feel very confident in your ability to perform well in the job for which you are applying. You need to show that you have masses of experience in the short time that you have been a SHO and that you have made a great effort to get to know the new hospital, unit and ward in which you will be working. You need to stress repeatedly during your answers that you feel 'entirely confident that you would be able to perform the job appropriately', but bear in mind your answers must not be so aggressive as to sound 'cocky' or over-confident. If you really feel that the present post is the chance of a lifetime then by all means say so in the interview, since this will continue the air of 'cool professionalism with enthusiasm' which is so important in ensuring success.

You're really not sure if you want this job or not

This is an issue that I addressed in the second chapter of this book. There is simply no excuse for sitting in an interview for a job which you are not totally certain that you want. Of course, you *may* apply for a job and then withdraw prior to the interview. Even if you find yourself in the horrible situation that you are in front of the interview panel and then decide that you really do not want the job, then you should say so and explain your reasons why. The real catastrophe is when individuals do well in an interview, are offered the job and then decline the job a couple of days – or worse still – a couple of weeks later. This generates intense animosity on the part of interview panels who will then have to be reconvened in order to appoint another candidate. It will potentially wreck your career because word gets around that you have 'dropped out after appointment' and there is certainly a chance that your referees will be contacted and an explanation will be demanded as to why you have behaved in the way that you have. Therefore, if you are not certain that you want this job make sure that you are not in the interview in the first place!

'CRINGE' QUESTIONS

Medical interviews are different from many other sorts of interview. Some people see them as more challenging than the interviews which our colleagues in industry face, others see them as very much lighter than the gruelling interviews faced by professionals in other walks of life. For example, if you were being interviewed for a post outside the world of medicine you might find yourself being asked a series of rather curious questions, for example, 'what are your strengths?', 'what are your weaknesses?', or 'what was your greatest achievement'? These are questions which most medical students and doctors would not find easy to answer at the best of times and they sometimes, albeit infrequently, crop up in medical interviews. They usually come from a panel member who cannot think of anything better to ask and occasionally they come from the 'vicar's wife' figure on the panel. These are sometimes rather irreverently referred to as 'cringe questions'. They gain that name because not only will you cringe when the question is posed, but virtually every other member of the interview panel will also inwardly cringe with embarrassment. So you need to get through these questions as quickly as possible, whilst at the same time not saying anything incriminating. Most of us could offer a fair answer to the question 'what are your strengths?' and an answer such as 'I'm a hard worker, I'm enthusiastic in what I do and most people say that I am very easy to get on with' is perfectly adequate and is quite long enough.

Rather harder is framing an answer to the question 'what are your weaknesses'? On occasion I have heard candidates offer astonishingly foolish answers to this question which immediately exclude them from any chance of success in the interview. For example, statements such as 'well, sometimes I find it impossible to get out of bed in the morning', or, worse still, 'well, I think I have a tendency to upset the nursing staff on my ward' reveal commendable frankness, but are catastrophic in terms of securing success in the interview. I suggest that the only suitable answer for the 'weakness' question needs to be something which allows the rest of the panel to chuckle and get over their embarrassment quickly. A good answer might be 'I must admit that I am obsessively punctual and completely intolerant of sloth', ideally delivered with a wry smile around the table. This sort of thing allows everybody on the panel to relax again.

As regards your 'greatest achievement', then few of us would feel that anything that we have done in medicine really rates as 'our greatest achievement'. If, however, you single-handedly ran a paediatric surgical unit in the middle of deepest Africa during your student elective period, then it might be reasonable to say so at this point. If you do not have an obvious medical achievement which is breathtaking, it is often better to retreat to a rather endearing answer and reply with something like 'being awarded my 50 m swimming certificate at the age of five'. Or 'receiving an invitation to give a solo organ recital in the local cathedral, following a successful school concert'.

'GOOGLIES'

Sometimes an interview panel member will throw a very unexpected and rather difficult question at you. It may be a confusing question or may seem to be needlessly aggressive. They are doing this for a reason and that is simply to see whether you are able to spark and cope when put under a bit of pressure. These questions are sometimes referred to as 'googlies'. It does not happen very often but you need to be prepared for the sort of question that goes 'I see that you have just spent 6 months working in Sunnydale accident and emergency unit. Everybody knows that that unit is totally useless and should be closed down forthwith. Don't you agree'? Remember that the other interview panellists will be surprised at hearing a question like this from one of their colleagues and therefore this can work to your favour. The interest of the interview panel will suddenly have been aroused and you can maintain their interest by being equally robust in your answer which might be along the lines of 'no, I totally disagree. I am aware of the rumours circulating regarding the Sunnydale casualty service but having worked there very recently I find these stories astonishing. They are totally unfounded. Furthermore, I would suggest that some of the work practices which we employ at Sunnydale are streets ahead of the services offered at comparable units. I think that the people making these criticisms should come and spend some time with us and see exactly what they could learn from the set-up at Sunnydale'.

You may get other questions that are less aggressive but equally likely to fox the unwary candidate. For example, 'if the centre of Birmingham were hit by a nuclear bomb tomorrow and all the hospitals at which you have been working during the past 5 years were destroyed, how would you rebuild them? Would it be one huge hospital or several small ones'? Obviously, there is no right or wrong answer to this sort of question but panels will be genuinely interested in your view. Any sort of well thought out plan to redevelop health services in Birmingham would be an acceptable answer. A bad answer would be something along the lines of 'well, I don't really know – I've never really put much thought into how hospitals function. I wouldn't be able to plan for a project like that'. This sort of feeble answer lacks enthusiasm and lacks sparkle.

HANDLING THE 'VICAR'S WIFE' PANEL MEMBER

You may well be asked questions by the lay member of the panel. It is an unfortunate fact that most of the other members of the interview panel will be rather less interested in the questions that come to you from this individual and probably less interested in your answers. Therefore, your answers need to be polite, enthusiastic but very much to the point. For example, if it says on your CV that you write children's books in Welsh then it is almost a running certainty that the lay member of the panel will want to spend some time talking to you about this. You need to be focused and crisp in your answers. This is because although it may be of great personal interest to you that you have achieved such literary success in Wales, it will not, however, be of any great interest to the rest of the interview panel. Your answers will give little clue as to whether you are or are not capable of doing the medical job for which you have applied. So you need to smile, be polite but keep your answers relatively short when it comes to the lay member of the panel. Remember all the time that you are trying to show 'cool professionalism with enthusiasm' and that 'cool professionalism' means professionalism as a medic not as a children's author. In your answers aim to keep coming back to your great enthusiasm for the medical subject for which you are applying. Avoid at all costs starting a mini-lecture on a non-medical subject to which you devote your spare time.

HILL WALKING AND MOTORBIKES

On your CV there will be a section headed 'interests' and towards the end of the interview one or other member of the panel will ask you something about your hobbies. The guiding principle here is similar to the principle which must be adopted when handling the 'vicar's wife' in that you need to be aware that there is a risk of becoming involved in a rather lengthy and inappropriate, discussion on diverse aspects of hill climbing, mountaineering equipment and so on. This may be of interest to the odd member of the panel that knows something about the sport, but will be of virtually no interest to any other member of the panel, all of whom will be getting bored at this stage in the interview. Therefore, if you are an enthusiastic hill walker or motorcyclist it is perfectly reasonable to say so, perhaps commenting in a sentence or two on the problems faced by the British motorcycle industry in the face of competition from the Japanese. However, do not get bogged down in this, since it is not what you are in a medical interview for. You can save that sort of discussion for the celebratory beer once you are successful after the interview.

ANY QUESTIONS FOR THE PANEL ... ?

In the same way that you can predict the opening questions in a medical interview, you can guarantee what the final question will be. The chairman of the panel will look at his colleagues and then will turn to you and will say something along the lines of 'well, that is all the questions that we have for you, I wonder if you have any questions for us'? What in fact the chairman of the panel is saying is that in their opinion the panel feel that the interview is now at an end. They wish to see the back of you and start on the next candidate. All of them are probably hoping that you will not have 'any questions for the panel'. Moreover, if you do have questions which you want to put to the panel now is not the right time to do it. You should have done it before the interview and if you have overlooked anything then you should sort it out afterwards.

I suggest therefore that there is only one suitable answer to this question and that is something along the lines of 'thank you but no. I have had the chance of meeting several members of the panel in advance of this interview and all my questions have been answered. Thank you'. And at that point you shut up. Somebody will then stand up and show you the way to the door. That is the time to leave.

AFTER THE INTERVIEW

chapter 5

THE JOB OFFER

If all has gone according to plan then a short while after the interview is finished the chairman of the panel will come out of the interview room and will invite you to 'come back in'. Almost always – but not absolutely inevitably – this means that you are the successful candidate and effectively means that you have got the job. Resist the urge to start hugging your fellow candidates at this stage, most of whom will suddenly feel an intense dislike towards you. Smile sweetly and try to look sympathetically towards the other candidates before smiling in a professional manner at the chairman of the interview panel and re-entering the room.

You will be invited to sit down and the chairman of the panel will announce something along the lines of 'we are delighted to be able to offer you the job'. Strictly speaking, the chairman of the interview panel has just made a significant error of protocol since in fact interview panels do not 'offer jobs', they simply make recommendations to the Trust Board of the hospital or to the regional postgraduate dean regarding who should be appointed. Only in exceptional circumstances, however, is the individual who is recommended by the interview panel not the person eventually selected for the job by the hospital. You should continue to retain a professional air and should thank the panel and agree that you will accept the job. A word of warning is necessary here since in the excitement of the moment it is very easy to make a mistake and announce that you will not just accept the job, but readily also accept all the unsatisfactory aspects of the job which you read about in the job description but chose to ignore up until this point. You might be better placed to thank the interview panel and announce that you will 'look forward to receiving their formal offer in the next day or two'. The reason why I advise a cagey approach at this point is that it is during the time between the interview and formally accepting the offer of employment that you may need to negotiate certain aspects of the post. This tends to be far more important at consultant level than at senior house officer (SHO) or specialist registrar level. You may now return home, or, as is sometimes the case, accept an invitation to go out for a beer with the interview panel, but whatever happens you can look forward to receiving a written letter offering you the job during the next few days.

NEGOTIATION

Negotiation at this stage may be all important. Remember that this is the first stage in the job application process at which you are in a position of power. You must not abuse that power since an aggressive negotiation style will go down very badly with your future colleagues and the worst case scenario is they will simply withdraw their offer of a job and will reconvene the panel with a view to appointing somebody different. You must therefore proceed with any negotiation with quiet diplomacy and tact, but at the same time, be confident about what you want to achieve.

SALARY

The most frequent source of negotiation is salary. In general terms individuals moving up the junior hospital doctor ladder should not take a drop in salary. Some appointees have successfully argued that their new salary should be greater not just than their previous basic salary, but that the new salary should be greater than previous basic *plus* payments for additional duty hours. Some hospitals are more easily won over on this point than others, but whatever the view of a given hospital, you should aim not to accept a drop in your annual basic salary.

The one important exception to this principle is when you move from the end of the specialist registrar ladder to consultant grade. At this point in the career ladder, there is no formal agreement to protect an individual doctor's salary and it is theoretically possible to lose out. For example, an individual on the top point of the specialist registrar scale, who was receiving a generous number of additional duty hour payments, might find that they are appointed to the bottom increment of the consultant salary scale and subsequently find themselves on a lower salary. This should be resisted and mindful of the unfair nature of such a move, most hospitals adopt a strategy as follows.

Individuals moving from a specialist registrar (or senior registrar) post into a consultant graded post will receive one incremental salary point up to a maximum of two increments on the consultant salary scale, for demonstrating that they have one or more of the following attributes:

1 They are over the age of 35 at time of appointment.
2 They hold a higher degree, i.e. MD or PhD.
3 They have been in a senior registrar appointment for more than 2 years before promotion to a consultant post.

4 They have previously worked as a locum consultant in their chosen speciality.

These four points are known as the 'unwritten rules' since they do not exist in any generally agreed form nor in any official document. They are applied by a large number of hospitals but *not by all* and there is very little you can do to enforce the application of these unwritten rules, except negotiation and attempts at gentle persuasion of your future managers. Bear in mind that this issue is now less relevant following the demise of the senior registrar grade. Nevertheless, senior specialist registrars who have been in post for several years may try to draw attention to these rules.

WITH WHOM TO NEGOTIATE

Negotiation after the interview and before taking up the offered post, is unlikely to be relevant to most junior doctors. It is, however, often important for new consultants. Discussion of salary should ideally take place with the chief executive of the hospital in which you will be working. There are very few other individuals, with the possible exception of the director of personnel, who have enough power to select the incremental start point of your new salary. You can seek the support of your new colleagues, but it is the managers who will ultimately decide. Remember that most hospital chief executives will be very willing to meet newly appointed consultants, especially so if they were not involved with the appointments process. It is entirely reasonable to request a meeting with this person very shortly after a successful interview. Issues such as salary and relocation expenses may be raised at this meeting.

Negotiation about other aspects of your job can often be better done with the clinical director of your new unit or the medical director of the hospital in which you will be working. It is up to these individuals to ensure that you have an adequate office with a reasonable amount of space and also proper secretarial support. The level of secretarial support will vary from one job to the next but if you are primarily based in a single hospital, perhaps spending no more than a half or one day out per week, you should expect to have the services of a full-time secretary. Many hospital managers now view this as an unreasonable luxury but nevertheless it is what you should aim for.

New consultants may feel that there are other aspects of the post which they want to negotiate. For example, if you feel that the job description is totally unreasonable in its demands and expectations, then the time between the offer of the job and your formal acceptance is one possible time to negotiate. Bear in mind, however, that it is often easier and less inflammatory to actually change your pattern of work once you have been performing according to the original job description for a period of several months. Excessively pushy negotiation and obstruction prior to accepting the job offer may simply mean that your future colleagues turn against you and decide to offer the job to someone else.

WHAT IF YOU WEREN'T SUCCESSFUL?

In my opinion there is no such thing as 'interview practice', at least not in front of a genuine panel. In the previous sections of this book I have urged that you obtain your practice in a mock interview situation with friends and colleagues. The real interview is inevitably a stressful occasion which requires a lot of investment of time and emotion if you are to be successful. Nevertheless, at times in your career you may fail to get the job that you want and this can be extremely distressing as well as giving rise to a loss of self-confidence. Try to make the best of a bad job and use the experience of an unsuccessful interview as a sort of tool to help you be more successful next time.

Most members of an interview panel are very happy indeed to speak in general terms about reasons why you were not selected for a job. Remember, however, that the deliberations of an interview panel are totally confidential, so they will not be able to discuss specific issues relating to exactly what was said behind closed doors. All the same, most members of a panel welcome a quiet approach some days after the interview to ask perhaps 'were there any questions which I handled particularly badly?', or 'was there anything on my CV which the panel felt made me unsuitable or inadequately qualified for the job'?

If you know members of the panel particularly well it is also useful to tactfully enquire whether 'they would advise you to continue using the same referees'. It is surprising how often, once prompted with a question such as this, a member of the interview panel will make a gentle suggestion that you 'consider changing referee number two'. Act immediately if given important information such as this.

Do not immediately assume that failure in an interview is a 'black mark' on your record, neither should it be considered any form of failure. Often interview panels anguish at great length, deliberating between two and sometimes three names, all of whom they would very much like to appoint to their job and feel rather regretfully that there is only one job to offer. Sometimes one member of the panel is despatched from the interview room after the result has been announced in order to offer comfort to the unsuccessful candidates. Try not to feel particularly aggrieved if at this stage you are told it was 'within a millimetre', or 'if only we had two jobs you would have got the second one'. It is very easy to retort that 'a miss is as good as a mile', but instead you should bite your lip and be encouraged by these warm comments.

CONCLUSION

chapter 6

This book contains a lot of information that I believe will be useful for junior doctors and also relatively senior doctors in applying for the next post in their career progression. Bear in mind that it represents one style of dealing with a job application and the process of being interviewed. The style which I have described may not suit everybody and if you feel that it would not suit you then do not use it. Do not try to pretend that you are someone other than yourself in the interview and do not try to answer questions in a way that seems somehow unnatural to you just because you think you are giving 'the right answers'.

Remember the important key messages stressed elsewhere in this book.

1 Make absolutely sure that you spot the advert in the first place.
2 Find out as much as you can about the interview panel before the interview.
3 Do not find yourself sitting in an interview for a job that you are not absolutely certain that you want.
4 Throughout the interview remember to try and give an impression of 'cool professionalism with enthusiasm'.
5 Aim to show the interview panel not just that you are 'right for the job' but also that the job is right for you *at this stage in your career*.

If you are unsuccessful do not assume that there is no hope for you and that you are an abject failure. You may have been ranked a close second behind a future Nobel prize winner.

Good luck! There is always an unpredictable side to medical interviews and a degree of luck as well as a great deal of skill is needed. The author of this book cannot, of course, accept any responsibility whatsoever if things do not work out. Equally, do not blame the author if you find yourself being unexpectedly successful in obtaining jobs that you had not really intended to get!

INDEX